Alpha Lipoic Acid

NATURE'S SUPREME
ANTIOXIDANT

Rita Elkins, M.H.

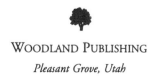

WOODLAND PUBLISHING
Pleasant Grove, Utah

1998
Woodland Publishing
P.O. Box 160
Pleasant Grove, UT
84062

CONTENTS

Introduction   5

Alpha Lipoic Acid: A Definition   6

A Brief History of ALA   7

Why Alpha Lipoic Acid is Important   8

The Power of Antioxidants   11

The Case for ALA Supplementation   11

Why ALA is the Perfect Antioxidant   15

ALA and the Treatment of Disease   17

Forms   23

Usage   24

Safety   24

Primary Applications of Alpha Lipoic Acid   25

Conclusion   25

Endnotes   27

INTRODUCTION

When a health supplement makes headlines on the five o'clock news and is chosen for Peter Jennings's copy script, you can be assured that it presents some remarkable therapeutic possibilities. Recently, Jennings very aptly described a remarkable experiment showing the wretched conditions of rats who had been fed a diet totally deficient in vitamin E. The rats were severely emaciated and debilitated. When given alpha lipoic acid, the rats returned to full health even though no vitamin E was replenished through nutritive sources. The implications of this laboratory test are profound. By giving these rats a compound called lipoic acid, existing stores of vitamin E that the body was unable to use were regenerated and given new life. The thought arises that if a compound can work to reactivate vitamin E within the body, what else can it do?

Alpha lipoic acid, a vitamin-like antioxidant which has been used in Europe for some time, is emerging as a much more impressive therapeutic agent and free-radical scavenger than previously assumed. Recent clinical tests have strongly suggested that its ability to halt some degenerative diseases, the oxidative process of aging and to actually restore the health of diseased organs is impressive, to say the very least. Moreover, it has the unique ability to make up deficits of vitamin E or C and may be one of the best treatments to recently emerge for diabetics.

Alpha lipoic acid—also referred to as ALA or thioctic acid—is considered more potent than vitamins E and C and even coenzyme Q10 by some health-care experts who are extolling its ability to protect cells from oxidation. Unlike other antioxidants, this compound has properties that make it superior in that it appears to be able to replace certain nutritional supplements, potentiate others, and actually inhibit the tissue deterioration we associate with so many diseases. Moreover, it is both fat and water soluble, enabling it to protect both lipid and aqueous cell structures.

While this supplement has been available for some years, it was not until 1988 that it emerged as an antioxidant powerhouse able to confer protection from free radicals both inside and outside the cell. Recent data shows that its properties are surprisingly impressive. It may be the most valuable antioxidant discovered to date.

ALPHA LIPOIC ACID: A DEFINITION

ALA can be defined as an antioxidant compound that is synthesized in the body in extremely small amounts. However, it must also be supplied from food or supplement sources to augment intrinsic supplies. It is a vitamin-like substance that contains sulphur and plays a vital role in energy reactions in mitochondrial electron transport. This function is intrinsically related to the metabolism of glucose into energy.

COMMON NAMES: ALA, thioctic acid, and lipoic acid.
CHEMICAL STRUCTURE: Similar to octanoic acid, ALA is comprised of a 6,8-dithiolane octanoic acid and a 1,2 dithiolane-3-valeric acid or a 1,2-dithiolane-3-pentanoic acid.[1]
PHARMACOLOGY: Alpha lipoic acid is a disulfhydryl coenzyme that converts to dihydrolipoic acid once inside cellular structures.

Dihydrolipoic acid is considered even more powerful free radical deactivator than the original acid. Dr. Lester Packer, a leading authority on ALA and professor of molecular and cell biology at the University of California at Berkeley, believes this particular attribute helps to make ALA the most effective antioxidant available. ALA appears to have the ability to deactivate both hydroxyl and single-oxygen free radicals. In addition, its dihydrolipoic form neutralized peroxyl and peoxynitrite free radicals. This latter type of oxidation is considered particularly damaging in that it contains both oxygen and nitrogen-based free radicals.2

FOOD SOURCES: Liver, yeast, spinach, organ meats, broccoli, red potatoes, and red meat.

BIOAVAILABILITY (degree of cellular absorption): When orally ingested, ALA is not compromised in the gastrointestinal tract or the liver.

A BRIEF HISTORY OF ALA

While numerous studies have been conducted on ALA confirming its positive effect on metabolic processes, recent, rather startling clinical tests support its ability to greatly enhance free-radical protection, slow the aging process, and guard against a number of degenerative diseases. Like DHEA, melatonin, and glucosamine, ALA is emerging as a biochemical compound capable of remarkable therapeutic actions.

Discovered in the 1930s, ALA was subsequently isolated during the 1950s. Originally classified as a vitamin, it was later categorized as an essential coenzyme in 1951 when scientists discovered that it was intrinsically involved in the energy processes of cell mitochondria. It was not until 1988 that scientists learned of its powerful antioxidant action. In addition, the fact that this antioxidant was both fat and water soluble made it even more impressive.

European practitioners have used ALA to treat the type of peripheral nerve damage associated with diabetes for over 20 years. German doctors routinely prescribe ALA for diabetic neuropathy, a fact of which very few American diabetics are aware. Dr. Lester Packer's work with ALA at the University of California in Berkeley has resulted in some remarkable findings that support the notion that ALA supplementation may benefit not only diabetics, but people with HIV as well. Its protective properties are unlike any other antioxidant compound. Recently, major national news organizations have featured ALA and its extraordinary properties on news broadcasts, suggesting that it may be the most powerful, versatile, and effective antioxidant discovered to date. Research on the compound continues at this writing.

WHY ALPHA LIPOIC ACID IS IMPORTANT

Virtually each and every day, most of us are exposed to a number of toxic substances—auto exhaust, tobacco smoke, pollution, preservatives, and additives continually assault our biocellular systems. In addition, diseases like diabetes, increased cholesterol levels, and just the pitfall of aging increase our risk of developing degenerative disease. The aging process can actually be accelerated by the presence of free radicals. Consequently, premature tissue breakdown can occur resulting in all kinds of ailments. In addition, despite our best efforts, our environment will continue to surround us with potentially harmful pollutants which all contribute to the creation of free radicals.

Certainly, there are several things we can do to minimize our health risks, including exercising, eating nutritiously, and not smoking. Unfortunately, these measures are rarely enough to substantially decrease our risk of certain degenerative diseases or of getting old before our time. While supplementing our diets with vitamins and minerals is strongly recommended, certain remarkable, natural substances such as alpha lipoic acid that have recently come to the forefront of scientific research.

Free Radicals: Cellular Culprits

Free radicals are molecules containing unpaired electrons. Unpaired electrons often cause a molecule to become unstable. In order to stabilize, they steal electrons from stable molecules, thus assaulting and altering healthy molecules. Free radicals bind to cell structures, causing damage and genetic change. They can initiate biological changes which can result in the formation of tumors, the hardening of arteries, the loss of skin elasticity, wrinkling, and organ failure. A free radical can destroy a protein, an enzyme, or even a complete cell. To make matters worse, free radicals can multiply through a chain-reaction mechanism resulting in the release of thousands of these cellular oxidants. When this happens, cells can become so badly damaged that DNA codes can be altered and immunity can be compromised.

Why Free Radicals are Dangerous

Even the very act of breathing creates these reactive chemical structures. To make matters worse, because our generation, more than any other, is exposed to a number of potentially harmful environmental substances, free-radical formation can reach epidemic proportions. Some of the more dangerous substances containing free radicals include:

- cigarette smoke
- smog
- x-rays
- gamma radiation

- pesticides
- car exhaust
- ultra-violet light
- rancid foods

- herbicides
- certain fats
- alcohol
- stress
- poor diet

- certain prescription drugs
- some food/water supplies

Contact with a free radical or oxidant on this scale can create cellular deterioration, resulting in cancer and heart disease. Tissue breakdown from this "oxidative stress" can also occur which contributes to aging, arthritis and whole host of other degenerative conditions. "Through free radical reactions in our body, it's as though we're being irradiated at low levels all the time. They grind us down."[3]

Unfortunately, because of the damage free radicals cause within our cellular structures, many of us will die prematurely from one of a wide variety of degenerative diseases. Free-radical damage has been associated with over 60 known diseases and disorders. Free radicals are responsible for a whole host of ills and ailments. If we could neutralize their damaging effects more effectively, we could immeasurably improve not only our longevity but the quality of our lives.

The Oxidative Downside of Exercise

As beneficial as it is, exercising can initiate the release of free radicals within our cellular systems. Aerobic exercising produces oxidation products. Many of these are not neutralized by our internal safety mechanisms and an overload can occur. Supplementing the diet with efficient antioxidants is highly recommended for everyone, but especially for those who exercise on a regular basis. ALA is particularly beneficial when it comes to the oxidation caused by exercise because it not only scavenges the oxidants left behind, it also helps to convert carbohydrates, fatty acids, and protein to ATP or energy needed to drive muscle movement.

THE POWER OF ANTIOXIDANTS

Potent substances called antioxidants scavenge for dangerous free radicals and so afford us the best prospect for disease prevention, toxin protection, and sustained longevity and vigor. According to many experts, making sure we arm our cellular systems with adequate supplies of antioxidants should be our first health priority.

"It has now been established that more than 60 human diseases involve free-radical damage, including cancer, heart disease and the acceleration of the aging process. All that you really need to know is that your body is under constant free-radical attack, and that you need to keep your antioxidant defenses strong."[4] Some of the most common of free-radical scavengers or antioxidants include:

- vitamin E
- vitamin C
- vitamin A/beta carotene
- coenzyme Q10
- selenium

While all of these are excellent cellular protectants, ALA is commonly excluded from antioxidant lists and may well be the most extraordinary free-radical scavenger of all.

THE CASE FOR ALA SUPPLEMENTATION

Because the small amounts of ALA produced by the body are bound to mitochondrial structures, very little of the acid is left over for other protective actions. While it is true that ALA is not technically considered an essential nutrient because it is produced within the body, it is only produced in trace amounts. Ironically, very few of us are aware that ALA supplementation may be just as critical to our well-being as more commonly used vitamins are. Unfortunately our bodies do not produce enough ALA to enable the compound to be utilized to its fullest antioxidant potential. For this reason, supplementation is more than warranted. Consider the following two reasons strongly suggesting that ALA supplementation makes good sense.

ALA Production Declines with Age

Frequently the oxidative stress caused by free radicals results in what we refer to as "the aging process." While aging is inevitable, many of us hasten its outcome by not protecting ourselves, hence, we age prematurely. The early onset of wrinkling, arthritis, circulatory disorders, diabetes, heart disease, and hardening of the arteries can result from free-radical damage that could have been minimized by consistently taking strong antioxidants like ALA.

Dr. Richard Passwater, author of *Cancer Prevention and Nutritional Therapies* states, "[Antioxidants] may be much more important than doctors thought in warding off cancer, heart disease and the ravages of aging—and, no, you may not be getting enough of these nutrients in your diet."[5]

ALA supplies, like human growth hormone, DHEA, melatonin, and coenzyme Q10 decrease with age.[6] This happens because the body's ability to synthesize these compounds declines, therefore food sources that contain ALA become even more important. Interestingly, the lack of every one of these compounds has been associated with the aging process, a fact which implies that if we could replace levels of ALA and other biochemicals before aging occurs, the process could be significantly inhibited. In addition, Dr. Packer points out that because we are living longer, we have to deal with increased incidence of age-related diseases.

Diet Alone May Not Provide Sufficient ALA

Clearly, while diet modifications are invaluable, diet alone cannot provide the kind of physiological defense the body requires to inhibit these free radicals before they cause biological harm. While there is no way to escape free-radical exposure, we can minimize their potential cellular destruction by reducing their numbers. Look at the types of foods that contain ALA. Liver, kidneys, spinach, red meat, and broccoli are certainly not the most popular foods most of us routinely consume. Even if we attempted to eat more ALA-containing foods, how many of us could sustain such a diet over a long period of time? Studies show that many of us are not even getting enough of what most consider more appealing foods, such as fruit, even though we may think we are. "The USDA conducted a study in which they collected dietary information over the course of the year for four independent days. In that study 20 percent of the adult women had no fruit or juice for four days, and about 45 percent had no citrus fruit or citrus fruit juice in four days."[7]

Only 9 percent of our population eats enough fruits and vegetables on a consistent basis. Unquestionably, most of us are not getting enough vitamin C and flavonoid compounds from our diets. Foods that are rich in vitamin E and selenium may also be lacking. Many of us neglect to eat enough whole grains, eggs, and other foods that contain natural supplies of vitamin E. In addition, it is important to remember that modern farming techniques, premature harvesting of fruits and vegetables, indefinite cold storage, freezing, canning, and cooking may denature food of its vitamin and coenzyme content. Because we know that diseases are often nothing more than nutritional deficiencies, we must make adequate supplementation a priority if we want to enhance our longevity.

Generally, we have failed to consume enough fresh fruits and vegetables on a consistent basis, suggesting that diet alone may not be enough to maintain optimal health and wellness. Clearly the diet guidelines provided by the RDA (Recommended Daily Allowance) fail to address the notion of optimal health or the fact that when we age or are fighting illness, our nutrient requirements dramatically escalate. ALA is contained in foods many of us find unappealing like liver, spinach or red meat. Obviously, for us, ALA food sources will be scarce and we may concede that supplementation is a good idea.

Symptoms of an ALA Deficiency:

Lab tests have found that when a deficiency of ALA occurs in animals, symptoms such as brain atrophy, reduced muscle mass, excess lactic acid production, or failure to grow and develop may result.[8] (Note: Tests have found that conditions like diabetes, cardiovascular disease, and liver disease can cause ALA depletion.[9])

Benefits Associated with ALA Supplementation

- reducing risk of cancer
- affording superior protection against toxins and pollutants
- inhibiting cellular mutation and HIV replication
- preventing premature aging and degenerative diseases like cataracts and senile dementia
- decreasing tissue damage in cases of heart attack or stroke
- reversing liver disease
- boosting the burning of glucose
- preventing diabetic neuropathy
- improving muscle strength
- anti-aging action
- protecting against extracellular LDL cholesterol
- improving memory

WHY ALA IS THE PERFECT ANTIOXIDANT

Dr. Lester Packer, who is considered one of the most informed ALA experts in the world, calls lipoic acid the ideal antioxidant because it can 1) scavenge free radicals of all kinds in both fat- and water-based cell structures; 2) rapidly assimilate and absorb into cells; 3) boost the action of other protective compounds; 4) chelate free meal ions; and 5) promote normal cell replication.[10] The following discusses why ALA has these remarkable properties.

ALA is Both Fat and Water Soluble

The fact that ALA is both fat and water soluble makes it a superior free-radical scavenger. In other words, it can protect both lipid and aqueous cell parts from free-radical damage. This dual solubility offers excellent cellular protection in that it can easily transport across cell membranes affording oxidant protection both outside and inside cell structures. The ability to become soluble in both mediums enables ALA to freely move throughout all cell parts, scavenging for free radicals in a way that is much more effective than other antioxidant compounds. For example, while vitamin C is a good antioxidant, it is strictly water soluble and only affects cell interiors. On the other hand, vitamin E is only fat soluble, which means that it affects only the lipid portion of cell structures or the membrane, leaving other areas unprotected.

ALA, Vitamin E, and Vitamin C: Perfect Synergy

One of the most exciting properties of ALA is its ability to interact with vitamin E and C, helping to not only conserve their stores but also to potentiate their actions. Dr. Packer found a most fascinating "recycling" relationship between vitamin E and C.[11] The presence of one enables the other to exert twice the antioxidant power. Taking ALA protects cells from the loss of vitamin E. ALA can increase cellular levels of these vital antioxidant compounds.

Lipoic Acid: Its Relationship to Glutathione

Cellular glutathione is produced in the body and, like other antioxidants, works to neutralize free radicals. Trying to artificially boost glutathione levels has been difficult, and while oral glutathione supplements are available, they must go through the gastrointestinal route before entering the blood stream. Unfortunately, little glutathione actually survives the digestive process. Consequently cellular levels are not significantly increased by oral supplementation.

Dr. Packer reports that supplementing ALA helps to regenerate glutathione, thereby providing extra cellular protection.[12] ALA allows glutathione levels to increase from within the body, an action which is particularly beneficial for anyone suffering from AIDS. Recent studies reveal that glutathione plays an intrinsic role in T-lymphocyte cell activity.[13] The ability of people suffering from HIV to transport glutathione into the cell is compromised; therefore, oxidative damage is accelerated. Because increasing dietary sources of glutathione does not significantly remedy this deficiency, the role of ALA is particularly crucial. It works in perfect tandem with glutathione to guard cells.

ALA Deficiency Can Impair Other Antioxidant Protection

Studies suggest that if the body becomes deficient in ALA, other antioxidant compounds may not work properly. This only makes sense in light of new evidence which reveals the very profound role ALA plays in boosting the activity of protective compounds like vitamin E. One thing is certainly evident—without

ALA, the mileage we get out of compounds like selenium and vitamin E is greatly limited. ALA dramatically extends the life and effectiveness of other vital antioxidant compounds. It must be understood that when antioxidants like vitamin E encounter free radicals, they become inactive. The presence of lipoic acid allows them to regenerate, thereby accomplishing a much greater level of cellular protection.

ALA Enhances Cellular Production of Energy

Dr. Packer believes that alpha lipoic acid also plays a vital role in the metabolic processes necessary to produce energy on a cellular level. ALA serves as a cofactor in the cellular process which converts carbohydrates, sugars, proteins, and fatty acids to energy.

If alpha lipoic acid were not present, cells would be unable to properly metabolize glucose in order to produce energy. As Richard Passwater puts it, this unique attribute makes ALA a metabolic antioxidant; a term which simply means that it can participate in the creation of ATP, while boosting the action of other antioxidant compounds. The biochemical role that ALA plays in the production of energy should not be underestimated. Boosting ALA levels through supplementation may help to enhance the production of energy, a function which is significantly compromised in individuals suffering from diabetes or other diseases.

ALA AND THE TREATMENT OF DISEASE

Diabetes and Blood Sugar

European medical practitioners have used ALA for decades to treat diabetic conditions and complications like diabetic neuropathy. Physicians at the Rostcok Sudstadt Clinic in Germany use higher-than-normal doses of ALA to reduce the symptoms of diabetic neuropathy. This serious side effect of diabetes causes peripheral nerve deterioration, which is a debilitating and painful condition. In some cases, ALA has been able to actually initiate a reverse in this condition. In addition, ALA helps to boost glucose uptake and in some cases has resulted in less insulin dependency.[14] German research supports the fact that using ALA resulted in a 50 percent increase in insulin-stimulated glucose dispersion in people suffering from adult-onset diabetes.

Experiments have confirmed the ability of ALA to increase the sugar-burning capacity of insulin, and to help reduce insulin resistance.[15] Insulin resistance is a major cause of adult-onset diabetes and is also closely linked to cardiovascular disease. In some people, obesity triggers this type of insulin resistance, causing sugar to stay in the bloodstream.

What is particularly relevant for anyone suffering from diabetes is that ALA has demonstrated its ability to prevent the type of protein modifications that can occur when blood sugar is elevated, called glycation.[16] This modification is responsible for creating a number of the very serious side effects that are associated with diabetes. Glycation occurs when elevated sugar levels in the blood react with body proteins found in the skin, arteries and veins, connective tissue, and myelin sheaths which protect the nerves. These reactions cause the formation of sugar-altered proteins which are, in essence, mutated proteins. It is the presence of these damaged proteins that causes so much tissue damage which manifests itself as atherosclerosis, retinal damage, kidney disease, slow wound healing, etc. ALA can help to reduce this process by facilitating the movement of sugar out of the blood and into cell structures where it belongs.[17]

Diabetics are especially prone to free-radical damage, but ALA can significantly reduce the oxidative damage caused by these radical molecules, helping to inhibit the development of many diabetic complications.[18] This fact alone makes ALA a very valuable therapeutic agent and should supplement the diet of diabetics.

Alzheimer's Disease

One of the most promising properties of ALA is the fact that it can protect brain tissue on a cellular level. German animal studies have found that ALA supplementation caused an improvement in the long-term memory of aged mice while younger mice showed no difference. What this finding implies is that ALA must help to reverse age-related memory impairment. It is assumed that the mechanism behind this action involves protecting brain cells from the kind of deterioration brought on by oxidation over time. Researchers believe that the chemical compounds found in ALA may help to treat a number of age-related neurological disorders.

Brain Tissue Protection

Researchers at the University of Rochester Medical Center found that ALA protected brain cells from certain hazardous chemicals. One of these was N-methyl-daspartate (or NMDA) which, when administered in excess, can cause neuron damage in the nervous system. Researchers involved in these trials reported that ALA may play a possible role in the treatment of acute or chronic neurological disorders such as Huntington's disease. It stands to reason that other neurological disorders may also respond to ALA therapy and while research with other diseases is lacking, supplementation may benefit anyone who suffers from Parkinson's disease, multiple sclerosis, and related disorders.

Cardiovascular Disease

We are all to aware now that LDL cholesterol plays a primary role in the development of cardiovascular disease. LDL cholesterol is particularly susceptible to free-radical damage. Free radicals cause cholesterol to snag onto artery walls creating a buildup of plaque. The accumulation of this fatty substance results in slower blood flow and eventually in heart attacks or strokes. When an artery becomes totally blocked or a piece of plaque breaks off and lodges in heart muscles or brain tissue, a heart attack or stroke occur.

Most cardiovascular emergencies are caused by a blockage which shuts off blood supply to tissue located either in the heart or brain, causing those areas to die from oxygen starvation. ALA can help to protect these tissues from the kind of damage a reduced oxygen supply causes. In addition, even when blood flow has been restored to these affected areas, a phenomenon called reperfusion, which results from increased free radical production, can cause even worse tissue damage than the original stroke or heart attack. Clinical trials involving animals have found that death from this type of tissue trauma was reduced by over 30 percent.

Atherosclerosis

The presence of LDL cholesterol in the bloodstream can lead to the formation of a deposit called arterial plaque which will eventually narrow vessels and may even break off causing a heart attack or stroke. Because vitamin E plays such a vital role in preventing this process called LDL oxidation, adding ALA to the mix only further potentiates this benefit. Remember, ALA and the compound it becomes on a cellular basis work to enhance the recycling of vitamin E. Therefore, taking ALA can make vitamin E much more effective and reusable. Instead of being "used up" after affording protection from LDL oxidation, vitamin E molecules are recycled, therefore their protective action can be exerted over and over again. In addition, ALA can help to protect LDL cholesterol from free radical damage itself. Laboratory tests have found that ALA can actually reduce blood cholesterol by 40 percent and LDL levels by

42 percent. What this amounts to is a very significant increase in the amount of oxygen supplied to both heart and liver tissue.[19]

Strokes

Dr. Packer's research also found that ALA can significantly increase the rate of survival in rats that had suffered a stroke if administered prior to the stroke. Because ALA goes into brain tissue, it can help to prevent the type of cellular damage which usually occurs when a portion of the brain becomes oxygen starved. Dr. Packer was part of a study where blood flow to the brain of test rats was restricted for 30 minutes, after which it was restored. Within 24 hours, 80 percent of the rats died. If they received lipoic acid, only 20 percent died; a result he refers to as the "most remarkable effect ever found in cerebral ischemia in a model system."[20] One of the main causes of death was due to the fact that glutathione levels dramatically dropped when blood flow was stopped to brain tissue. Even the administration of glutathione did not remedy this deficit. It was through ALA supplementation that glutathione levels increased, thereby lowering the mortality rate.

Cancer

Free radical damage can promote the activity of a certain cell protein called factor kappy-B (NF-kB). This protein works to promote inflammation and genetic changes that have been associated with the development of malignancies. In vitro studies at the University of California at Berkeley have found that when cells are bathed in ALA, this particular factor is inhibited, therefore, cell mutations cannot continue to replicate. This finding has significant implications for the type of protection we need to prevent ourselves from developing malignant cells. The type of genetic changes which accompany the formation of a cancerous tumor are inhibited by the presence of ALA.

Cataracts

Cataracts form when degenerative changes take place in the lens of the eye, causing the buildup of a cellular residue that compromises vision. In the case of cataracts, we are dealing with an aqueous environment or water-based tissue. It is important to remember that both beta carotene and vitamin E are lipid-based antioxidants that do not effect watery cell structures. Studies strongly suggest that ALA significantly boosts the presence of ascorbate, glutathione, and other protective enzymatic compounds in the eye, protecting against the formation of cataracts. In essence, ALA was able to restore not only glutathione but ascorbate reductase as well in the eye lens of test animals. When animals were given a cataract-forming compound, they all developed cataracts. When ALA was administered, 60 percent of the animals did not develop cataracts.[21]

HIV

One of the most surprising discoveries concerning ALA was that it can inhibit the replication of the HIV-1 virus by "sticking" to the viral DNA. In vitro tests found that ALA could completely inhibit the action of a certain gene in the AIDS virus which enables it to replicate. Moreover, ALA has also been reported to help normalize immune function and is especially beneficial for T-lymphocyte cells which are directly impacted by the HIV virus. Recent studies have found that AIDS patients who received ALA experienced a dramatic increase in glutathione and vitamin C. In addition, the type of destructive oxidation typical of the disease process declined in over half of the subjects studied.

Liver Regeneration

ALA has also been linked with better oxygenation of liver tissue and impressive detoxification properties. Some health practitioners recommend taking it in conjunction with silymarin to help stimulate liver tissue regeneration. In cases where metal poisoning has taken place, taking ALA with silymarin should be particularly effective in boosting the ability of the liver to detoxify. In addition, cirrhosis of the liver, which is caused by alcohol, also responds to ALA therapy. Silymarin has also demonstrated its remarkable ability to stimulate liver tissue growth and is highly recommended for anyone suffering from alcohol-related liver disease.[22]

Detoxification

ALA has been used to protect the liver from toxins and other pollutants such as heavy-metal compounds, including copper and iron, toxic metals like mercury and cadmium and when combined with vitamin E, can actually treat radiation exposure by protecting cells from the oxidation that radiation initiates.[23] ALA therapy has been used to treat children who were exposed to the radioactive fallout after the Chernobyl accident in Russia. It has been referred to as an impressive compound chelator capable of extracting excess iron and copper from the bloodstream.[24] Silymarin, mentioned in the previous section, also has impressive liver detoxification properties again suggesting that using ALA in conjunction with silymarin may provide excellent liver support in cases of alcohol toxicity as well as other poisonous substances.

FORMS

ALA can be purchased in both tablet and capsule form. It works well when orally ingested in that it is easily assimilated through the walls of the gastrointestinal tract.

USAGE

Generally speaking, taking between 40 to 50 mg of ALA is considered a therapeutic dose for maintaining health, while doses in the 100 mg range are used for chronic conditions. Diabetics can take between 200 and 300 mg per day and even more if their physician feels it is necessary. AIDS patients can go over this dose, but must do so under the supervision of their physician. ALA therapy is a long-term treatment and is usually not associated with short-term results.

SAFETY

Generally considered safe, ALA has been used for over 20 years in Europe with no reported toxicity or adverse effects. It is well tolerated and assimilated through the stomach. Animal studies have found that doses over 400 to 500 mg/kg of body weight can create some toxicity. This amount translates to dosages higher than most people would use as a preventative antioxidant compound. Children and pregnant or lactating women should not take this supplement. Anyone who is under the care of physician or has a serious medical condition should check with their doctor before using ALA. This supplement is considered safe if used as directed. ALA may interfere with vitamin B1 assimilation therefore anyone suffering from a thiamine deficiency, such as many alcoholics, should take a thiamine supplement in conjunction with ALA.

PRIMARY APPLICATIONS OF ALPHA LIPOIC ACID

- Aging
- AIDS
- Alcoholism
- Atherosclerosis
- Bell's Palsy
- Cataracts
- Cancer
- Cirrhosis
- Diabetes
- Diabetic Neuropathy
- Multiple Sclerosis
- Liver Disease
- Radiation Sickness or Exposure
- Memory/Alzheimer's Disease, Senile Dementia
- Stroke
- Huntington's Disease
- Parkinson's Disease
- Heavy-Metal Poisoning

CONCLUSION

ALA offers some of the most impressive antioxidant properties yet discovered. In addition, not only does it seem to afford superior protection against the free radicals that cause brain, heart, and liver damage, it boosts the protective action of other antioxidant compounds like vitamin E and Glutathione. It is remarkably versatile and due to the magnitude of its recently discovered properties, scientific research has been stepped up.

What makes it particularly appealing is that it is easily absorbed and can benefit both fat-based and water-based cell structures. This dual action makes ALA unique and incredibly effective as a cell-protectant. Because dietary sources of this nutrient are not what most of us consider foods we routinely eat, supplements are highly recommended. German medical practitioners have used ALA supplements for years in treating certain conditions and consider it safe. The therapeutic implications of ALA are striking, to say the very least, and make other antioxidants pale in comparison. Referred to by Dr. Packer as the "universal" antioxidant, this compound is not only powerfully protective, but certainly capable of cellular benefits which undoubtedly still remain unknown to modern medical researchers.

Supplementing our diet with what is perhaps nature's most powerful antioxidant is certainly paramount in protecting ourselves and our families from the ravages of aging and disease. It would seem only logical that the earlier we start using ALA supplementation, the better for our biocellular health, and all health is determined on a cellular level. While we anxiously await for the cure for cancer and other devastating diseases, we can arm our bodies with the most powerful protective nutrients available. Alpha lipoic acid is the compound of choice.

Dr. Packer's work and impressive track record in the field of antioxidants suggests that ALA supplementation is destined to become the most valuable therapeutic protocols we can utilize. In addition, as more scientific evidence presents itself, ALA supplementation may become one of the most remarkable health practices of the twenty-first century.

ENDNOTES

1. Lester Packer, Ph.D. et al., "Alpha lipoic acid as a biological antioxidant," *Free Radical Biology and Medicine*, 1995, 19: 227-250.
2. Ibid.
3. *New York Times*. (April 25, 1993).
4. *Time Magazine*. (April 6, 1992).
5. Richard A. Passwater Ph.D., *Cancer Prevention and Nutritional Therapies*, (New Canaan, Connecticut: Keats Publishing, 1993).
6. Packer, 227-50.
7. G. Block, University of Southern California at Berkeley.
8. Michael T. Murray, *Encyclopedia of Nutritional Supplements*, (Prima Publishing, Rocklin, California: 1996), 343.
9. V.E. Kagan, et al., "Dihydrolipoc acid: A Universal antioxidant both in the membrane and in the aqueous phase," *Biochem Pharmacol*, 1992, 44: 1637-49.
10. Packer, 229-250.
11. M. Podda, et al., "Alpha-lipoic acid supplementation prevents symptoms of vitamin E deficiency," *Biochem Biophys Res Commun*, 1994, 204: 98-104.
12. Han D. Tritschler, et al., "Alpha-lipoic acid increases intracellular glutathione in human T-lymphocyte Jurkat cell line," *Biochem Biophys Res Commun*, 1995, 207: 258-264.
13. R. Buhl, et al., "Systemic glutathione deficiency in symptom-free HIV-seropositive individuals," *Lancet*, 1989, 2: 1294-97. See also G.B. Corcoran et al., "Suppression of human immunodeficiency virus expression in chronically infected monocyte cells by glutathione, glutathione ester and N-acetyl cysteine," *Proc Natl Acad Sci USA*, 1991, 3: 986-90.
14. S. Jacob et al., "Enhancement of glucose disposal in patients with type-2 diabetes by alpha-lipoic acid," *Arzneim Forsch*, 1995, 45: 872-74. See also D. Elizabeth et al., "Stimulation of glucose uptake by the natural coenzyme alpha-lipoic/thioctic acid: participation of elements of the insulin signaling pathway," *Diabetes*, Dec., 1996, 45 (12): 1798.
15. S. Jacob, et al., "The antioxidant lipoic acid enhances insulin-stimulated glucose metabolism in insulin-resistant rat skeletal muscle," *Diabetes*, 1996, 45: 1024-29.
16. Y. J. Suzuki, et al., "Lipoate prevents glucose-induced protein modifications," *Free Radical Res Commun*, 1992, 17: 211-17.
17. Jacob, 1024-29.
18. A. Constaninescu, et al., "A-lipoic acid protects against hemolysis of human

erythrocytes induced by peroxyl radicals," *Biochem, Mol Biol Int,* 1994, 33: 669-679. See also P. J. Guillausseay, "Pharmacological prevention of diabetic micro angiopathy," *Diabetes Metabol,* 1994, 20: 219-28 and J.T. Greenamyre, et al., "The endogenous cofactors, thiotic and dihydrolipoic acid are neuroprotective against NDMA and malonic acid lesions of striatum," *Neuroscience Letters,* 1994, 171: 17-20.

19. R. Passwater, *Lipoic Acid: The Metabolic Oxidant,* (Keats Publishing, New Canaan, CT: 1996).

20. Interview with Dr. Lester Packer and R. Passwater in *Whole Foods Magazine*/Lester   Packer-Health Worldchttp://www.healthworld.com/LIBRARY/Article/passwater?PACER3 . HTM.

21. I. Maitra, et al., "Alpha-lipoic acid prevents buthionine sulfoximine-induced cataract formation in newborn rats," *Free Radical Biology and Medicine,* 1995, 18: 823-829.

22. R. Braatz, "The effect of silymarin on intoxication with ethionine and ethanol," *Braatz and Schneider,* 1976, op cit., 31-36.

23. Packer, *Free Radical Biology and Medicine,* 1995.

24. O. P. Tritschler, et al., "Thiotic (lipoic) acid: A therapeutic metal-chelating antioxidant?" *Biochem Pharmacol,* 1995, 50: 123-26.